LOSE WEIGHT THE HEALTHY WAY

by
Brandi Yeargain

Introduction:

We all reach that moment in our lives where we really aren't feeling all that great about how we look. There are many different bad ways to take care of this issue and good ways as well. Let's be honest, everyone's bodies are different and react to diets in a different way. There are fad diets that might work for a little while, but aren't really all that healthy for you and don't give your body what it needs to function properly. I am going to go over all of this throughout my book. My plan is to give you everything you need to know in order to diet the healthy way. This means you will not be hungry all day, you will slowly lose weight and in the end you will feel great inside and out. I reached this moment in my life about 5 years ago when I really wasn't feeling good about the way I looked. The bigger problem was that I wasn't feeling well either. I was starting to have stomach problems where I either had diarrhea or was vomiting. This is why I want you to learn the healthy way of losing weight, so that you won't do your body more harm than good. I was going to the gym and working my butt off and then went home and drank my water and watched those calories. I lost 25 pound and was so proud of myself. The problem with this was that I felt horrible doing it. I was tired and didn't really have enough energy to get through the day and I was constantly hungry. Let's fast forward 5 years where I learned how to lose weight the right way. I dropped another 17 pounds, I feel great and it was almost effortless because I was doing it the right way. If you are losing weight you need to be doing it the healthy way and you need to be doing it for the rest of your life.

Chapter 1:
Why Diets Fail

There are many reasons why the many diets' you have tried have failed; and I am going to tell you why. First things first, so many of these diets have you starving your body. You are only allowed so many calories a day, you can only eat 1 food or you can't eat one certain food. The problems with these diets are that you are taking away key vitamins and nutrients that your body needs in order to function the right way. Let's talk about the first one I mentioned, you are only allowed to eat a certain amount of calories a day. Most of us drop to 1500 calories on a diet. So here you are only eating 1500 calories and you are hungry. For the most part you have been good, at least until you get to after dinner and have eaten 1550 calories. This is where you convince yourself that you are already over by 50 degrees and the snack you have been craving all day will be fine as long as you only have a few bites and do 300 jumping jacks before bed. Why are you making yourself jump through so many loops to lose weight and why are you making yourself feel guilty for it? It's because you know you want to lose the weight but you want it to be easy and you want to go to bed feeling like you were actually fed throughout the day. I get it, and I couldn't agree with you more. You should not be hungry while you are on a diet. Period. Just because you are on a diet does not mean you have to walk around drooling over every little piece of food you see because you are starving yourself.

Elimination diets are just as bad because they are giving you one of more items that you cannot eat. Don't eat any chocolate and you can lose 30 pounds in a month. We all know this doesn't work because what do we want to eat? Yep you guessed it, Chocolate! Once you have it in your head that the one thing you can't eat is exactly what you want, there is no turning back. The problem with this diet is that if you do follow it and you happen to lose weight, when you are done that's the first thing you are going to reward yourself with so all of your hard work goes down the drain. It will be like a long lost friend you haven't seen in forever and absolutely need to get your hands on it.

Fake health foods are a culprit also. There are a few things that drive me crazy and this is one of them. There are so many companies ready to put "**HEALTHY**" on a bag of something they produce because people want healthy foods now. The thing is they don't have to be telling the truth for them to make money and frankly they don't feel bad about the lie they are telling you either. It just has to be a little bit of the truth in order for them to get away with it. For instance, if it say's healthy it could just mean it's 5 calories less than its competitor. If you look at the nutrition label and there are things in it that are unhealthy, odds are that new and improved snack is not a health choice. My main go to is that if it's in a box ready to eat, or has been processed it's not healthy.

Soy is one of these products also. Soy is nothing more than filler that is put into your food to make you feel full. Over 75% of soy is not picked from a plant but made in a lab. Anything that is made or processed in a lab is not good for you. In fact, soy has a ton of extra hormones that mess with your body. Women are having longer periods, and ovarian cysts because of all of the extra hormones that are being put into our foods. Men are also having testosterone problems and a lot of this can all be blamed on our foods that we are eating. This same idea goes a long with oils that have been produced in a lab and don't have anything-healthy much less natural in them. You have to be wary of foods that are labeled health foods because a lot of those are nothing more than a lie.

Vitamin water is something that is trying to be healthy but really just isn't. I would love to tell you that this is water that is good for you and has some flavor but I just can't. So here is this wonderful drink that calls itself water and healthy but then on top of it adds as much sugar as a soda does. These are the things I need you to open your eyes to, the hidden junk they are putting in items they call health food.

Fad diets are nothing more than something that is popular for the moment. People get on these diets and while they do drop the weight, they are starving their body, brain, bones and muscles in order to do it. The cabbage soup diet promises that you can lose up to 10 pounds in 7 days. The good thing on this diet is that if you are hungry you can eat all you want of the items that are on the list. The bad thing is the fact that you are starving your body of nutrition it really needs and the fuel you need to function through the day. People are complaining that they are feeling light headed and tired, well that's because you aren't giving your body what it needs in order to function properly. Also with all of the foods that you are allowed to eat on this diet, you will be spending more time in the bathroom than you will want to.

Juice cleanses are another one that worries me. You are getting your vitamins from this one that is true but you aren't eating anything to actually digest. With all those liquids, running to the bathroom will be your new sport. You see there is a reason why these diets don't last on the market that long. They just don't give your body what it needs to survive.

Diet supplements and that wonderful magic diet pill that works miracles are nothing more than empty promises. Let's be honest with ourselves, if we can lose weight fast and not have to really put any effort into it, it sounds like a good deal right. Well the problem with this is that there are always side effects to pills like these. First of all, the pills hype you up on a ton of caffeine and on top of that you have to drink 2 glasses of water with them so you aren't hungry. Here you are minding your own business bouncing off the walls and you are starting to feel bad. Why wouldn't you? You haven't eaten anything to keep your body going. It is running off of nothing more than that caffeine pill. You have no vitamins or nutrients for your body to run on. Do you know what happens when your body has no food in its system? It pulls it from your brain, bones and muscles. This is not the proper way to lose weight it just sounds good on paper because you don't want to work at it.

Chapter 2:
Know what your body needs

Your body needs a certain amount of vitamins, nutrients and minerals in order for it to have enough fuel for it to function the way it is supposed to. There are a number of things to make sure that your body gets. Of course some of those you need to keep at a minimum level. First we will look at your recommended daily amount of things that you need to keep at a minimum.

Total Fats- 30%
Saturated Fats- 8-10%
Trans fats- less than 1%
Cholesterol- less than 300 milligrams
MUFAS- up to 20%
PUFAS- up to 10%
Sugar- 25% for women and 32% for men.

It's important for you to keep all of these levels at or lower than the recommended daily intake. Now you also need to get your daily allotment of Vitamins, Minerals and nutrients. It's better if you are getting these from actual food instead of vitamins. The reason for this is simply because if an animal has eaten grains that were growing in a field, it makes it easier for your body to digest and absorb all of the nutrients you need. However, if you add vitamins on top of a balanced diet it is ok.

When you eat food that is natural, it is easily digested and all of the healthy vitamins and minerals give your body energy to move throughout your day. When you eat meat and vegetables you are able to process these foods and get the most from them because they are natural. These healthy foods are what you need to be making sure that you are getting enough of, each and every day so that you are feeding your brain, bones and muscles.

Cutting carbohydrates from your diet was the best new diet a few years ago but this is another diet that really drove me crazy. People are going around on low carbohydrate diets because it helps you lose weight. I don't blame them because it works, but it's not healthy. Your body needs carbs. You have been told that carbs are in breads, cakes, pastries and all of those wonderful sweet treats we all love. I feel like there is a large percentage of the world's population that is unaware that some vegetables are also carbs and they give your body energy. In fact, your body gets most of its energy from carbohydrates. So if you are cutting your carbs you are cutting your energy. Healthy carbs include corn, bananas, white potatoes, sourdough bread and green peas. Please enjoy your carbohydrates in order to give your body that wonderful energy boost it needs, just do it in moderation like everything else you put in your body.

Ok here is another one that is going to be a surprise. Your body needs fat. Your brain feeds off of it and if you are not getting enough in your body, it starts pulling fat from your brain. Let's not go crazy with this information you still need to keep it at a healthy amount but stop buying the low fat foods. These are not healthy for you. This is one of the other fake health foods that are just making people think they are eating healthy. Eat natural fats like bacon grease, extra virgin olive oil, coconut oil and avocado oil. Keep an eye out for the oils that have been produced by people instead of nature. These kinds of items sit in your gut and slowly digest instead of digesting quickly. This causes discomfort, gas and bloating. Here is a helpful list for your bad and good fats.

BAD FATS	GOOD FATS
CORN OIL SOYBEAN OIL SUNFLOWER OIL VEGETABLE OIL PALM OIL	ACOCADO OIL CANOLA OIL EXTRA VIRGIN OLIVE OIL NUT OILS NUT BUTTERS
BUTTER CHEESE LARD MARGARINE	FLAXSEED FATTY FISH PUMPKIN SEEDS SESAME SEEDS SUNFLOWER SEEDS WALNUTS
CHICKEN WITH SKIN HIGH FAT CUTS IN MEAT COMMERCIAL BAKED GOODS FRIED FOODS	BUTTER (GRASS FED COWS ONLY) EXTRA VIRGIN COCONUT OIL FLAXSEED OIL OMEGA-3 OIL

Chapter 3:
Sugar could be your enemy

Sugar is something that we all love and enjoy. However, it doesn't really love us back. It has been proven that sugar is more addictive than cocaine! We have it in our drinks and all of those delicious desserts we convince ourselves we deserve but it's also in all of our other foods that we don't even notice. Have you looked at a nutrition label lately? It's in everything. America is one of the worst nations when it comes to eating sugar. We put twice the amount of sugar in a recipe than is needed. The problem with sugar is that once it is eaten it sits in your stomach trying to be absorbed and leaves us with all of that stomach fat we hate so much. It's in beef jerky, bread, peanut butter, frozen fruit, crackers and so much more. Of course this makes lowering your sugar intake so much harder because it's other job is to give you cravings.

Its not all bad news when it comes to sugar though because there are natural sugars that you can take advantage of. You can eat as much fruit as you want and thoroughly enjoy it. Natural sugars come from fruit so it is time you start enjoying fruit. I have to be honest I am not a huge fan of eating fruit. I don't like to eat apples or bananas but I had to get over this little hump when I decided to take my health into my own hands. I found that my cheats are smoothies. All fruit that I froze myself so it didn't have added sugar. This is the way I feel like I have gotten a sweet treat without cheating and eating sugar. Honey is also ok to eat but still needs to be limited. The thing is, a person is supposed to have 25 grams of sugar a day of you're a woman and 32 if you are a man. Preferably less but up to these amounts. The problem with this is that most people drink sodas and juices, which have a ton of sugars. Just one soda can put you over your limit for the day. Eat as much natural sugar as you want, there is no need to calculate that sugar but I do want you to count the added sugar you eat in your diet. This is the one place I want you to be strict. I am not asking you to cut it from your diet completely but eat as little as you can and realize you get it in unwanted places like a slice of bread.

Sugar substitutes are one of the things that you really should be staying away from. They are not good for you. I don't care what the company trying to sell it to you says. They are manmade not nature made! They sit in your gut, add to your waistline and make you crave sugar. Basically they make you back slide on the diet you are trying to be good on. These fake sugars are trying to make you believe that you are being good to your body when actually you are just hurting it. That goes for all of the sugar free items also because they are all made with sugar substitutes. You need to be looking for "No Sugar Added" products. They have no added sugars including sugar substitutes. My favorite treat right now is Outshine popsicles, the **no added sugar** kind. They are real fruit and can be counted as a serving of fruit.

Sugar works in many ways to harm your body. It makes you gain weight, which is the main problem we are trying to solve, but it also gives bacteria in your body something to thrive on. Bacteria is fed by sugar, so if you are suffering from a stomach virus, urinary tract infection or any other kind of bacterial infection, the more sugar you are eating the worse this virus is going to get. Now in saying that, I want you to think about the last time you had a UTI and were told to drink cranberry juice. Inside that cranberry juice was upwards of 15% sugar! This was not only making your pain go down but also allowing the bacteria to grow and need those antibiotics to fight the infection even more.

So here we are at the point where it is up to you on whether or not you chose to cut your sugar in order to lose the weight. You would be amazed at how well you feel with just a little less sugar. This does mean some sacrifices. Sodas carry so much sugar it would be a good idea to cut those out of your diet and just go with some water. You can continue drinking your coffee but I do suggest cutting half of the sugar in that also. Just try your hardest to stay at the amount you are supposed to be at for the day (25 grams for women and 32 grams for men) and from there try to eat less and less each day. Don't forget if you get a major craving make a smoothie to help yourself out. The more natural sugars you are taking advantage of the easier this process is going to be. My go to snack for sugar cravings is frozen grapes or smoothies. Both of these make you feel like you are getting a treat when you are actually eating right.

Chapter 4:
My Diet Plan

Here we are the big moment you have been waiting for. This is the moment I tell you everything you need to know in order to grab this diet plan by the horns. This is the part that takes effort and struggle. If you follow the plan you will drop weight. After the first month it will be easy. It is starting the plan that is hard. It is hard because you are changing the way you eat, and think about food. I want you to be picky about what you stick in your mouth. I want you to be happy about the things you are eating and your weight as it drops. I'm not going to lie to you it will not be fast. It won't be fast because it shouldn't be fast. Hang in there and don't get discouraged. This is about looking great and feeling great.

Eat real Food
So here is the first step in my diet plan. You have to eat real foods. I don't want you buying boxed items like macaroni and cheese or hamburger helper. Stay away from the aisle that has all of these in it. If you are going to eat it, I want it being from real vegetables and fruits that you buy and chop up. Why is this so important? Well because natural foods are not processed and do not have a lot of extra additives in them. These are nothing more than fillers and fillers are our bodies' enemies. These are the things our bodies do not digest well and if we stop eating them our bodies process food the way they are supposed to. If your body can process the food easily it is not sitting in your gut turning into fat but it is being kicked out of your body once you have received all of the nutrients you need from it.

Limit your sugar intake
I know, I know I told you I wasn't going to have you stop eating a food. I'm not I am just asking you to cut it down to how much you are supposed to eat on a daily basis. I love sugar as much as you do but I can tell you I feel so much better now that I have cut most of the added sugar out of my diet. Start with baby steps because this one is going to be the hardest. If you drink multiple sodas a day

cut it down to 1 and measure out 8 ounces. This will also help if you are experiencing withdrawal symptoms. If you drink coffee with 2 tsp of sugar and flavored coffee creamer cut both of these in half. Write down the amount of sugar you are eating every day and by the end of the first week you need to be down to your allotted amount. Period! No excuses. After that see how little you can get away with until you are as low as 10 grams of sugar a day. Remember I don't count natural sugars that come from real fruit. Eat all the natural sugars from fruit that you want. You can go crazy with them. Just get away from the added sugar that is doing your body so much harm. I want you looking at nutrition labels so that you know how much sugar you are getting. Remember it is hiding in everything that is at your grocery store. If you buy a loaf of bread you are going to have to count that sugar intake when you eat a sandwich.

Drink mostly water

I want you drinking mostly water because it is easily digested and runs through your system. It keeps your kidneys healthy and works wonders for your skin. I had always heard that everyone needed to drink 64 ounces of water a day. It wasn't until I took my nutrition course that I found out that isn't quite right. To figure out how much water you should be drinking a day, take your weight and cut it in half. That is the amount of water you should drink a day. So if you are 200 pounds you need to be drinking 100 ounces of water a day in order to stay hydrated. This also works wonders when it comes to eating the right amount of food for your body. If you are drinking the amount of water you are supposed to, you won't be hungry enough to over eat.

Enjoy your food

Ok now that we have gotten all of the unhappy things out of the way, I want you to enjoy your food. Eat what you like and enjoy it. I don't want you going out and eating rice cakes because they are low in calories because you are going to want to cheat later. In saying that, you also need to make sure you have vegetables on your plate. I am a Texas girl and we all love our big portions of meat with a little bit of vegetables. However, your meat portion should be the size of your fist and two vegetables on your plate should be about the same size if not bigger. This makes sure your body is getting everything you need in a meal and are full afterword.

Enjoy your spices

At some point with all of the diet foods we were made to believe that our food had to taste like cardboard in order to lose weight and of course be healthy for you. Well I am here to tell you that it doesn't. Use your spices and make your food enjoyable. Your diet will not work if you are not enjoying the food that you are eating. Real natural herbs and spices are best but regular bottled dried ones work also. Either way your food will have some flavor and you will be happy eating it. So put the dry flavorless rice cake down and eat some real food with some real flavor! Use your spices as much or as little as you like, there is no reason to cut flavor when you are trying to be healthy.

Make Meal Plans

Each week sit down and make a plan of what you are going to eat throughout the week. Know what breakfast, lunch and dinner will be. This helps to cut out all of the unnecessary fast food nights. I know we all get busy working during the week and we just want something fast but the more you are making at home the healthier your body will be. Also you don't have to be rigid you can skip around. The point is you know what you are going to eat throughout the week and you have all of those items on hand. If you do have a night where you fail and go out to eat, make healthy choices. You know the fried chicken was fried get the grilled instead. Little baby steps everyday will help you to drop the weight. If you have a pizza night at your house, enjoy your pizza like normal but instead of 2 slices eat 1 slice and have a side salad. Think about how many calories, and fat you cut just by lowering the amount you eat by 1. You are still going to be full because you have a side salad to fill your stomach along with that amazing piece of pizza you have been wanting all week.

Shop a week at a time

Once a week go to the grocery store and make sure you have made a list and get everything on it. This will help to keep your grocery budget down also. Go through your pantry to make sure you have everything on your list that you need. Do not go to the grocery store when you are hungry. I know some of you can't do this next tip but please try to go without the kids because they have a wonderful way of making you buy all those sugary snacks we don't need. If you have to take them try to buy healthy snacks instead of items that are packed with sugar.

Use smaller plates

We are happy and feel fulfilled when our plates are full. You can still fill your plate just eat on a small one. This way when you fill it up it isn't as much as if you had a large plate in front of you that is full. Going along with the bigger plates, learn to stop eating when you are full. If you are full don't force yourself to finish off the food on the plate. Overeating is a big problem because all of us have been taught to finish the food on our plates. Start off with less and add more if you are still hungry so you don't feel bad about throwing food away. But I am going to say it one more time, stop eating when you are full.

Snacks

Eat snacks if you need them. I recommend smoothies (made at home with real fruit), frozen grapes or Outshine popsicles. These are my favorites because of the sugar content. They give me that sweet flavor I am looking for and fill the urge to sit down and eat an entire pint of ice cream. Also I mentioned grapes. It is more work but when you get home wash them and pick them off of the vine. Place them in a large bowl and set them on the table each night with dinner. Eat a few after you are done with your plate. Not only do they help with digestion they also get in an extra bit of fruit with your meal.

Chapter 5:
Your Weight Loss Journey

Before you begin you need to be ready to lose weight. It can't be because someone else wants you to be healthier; it has to be your goal. I cannot stress this enough, you have to be the one to want to lose the weight or you will fail. It's not going to be hard to follow this Diet plan but it will take persistence and it will change your life. This is not a 2-week plan; it is a rest of your life plan. I want you feeling great inside and out and I want you making the decision to be a healthier you.

Day 1 of your new diet, I want you to get a notebook and a measuring tape. Measure around your boobs/chest, your biceps, your waist, your hips, thighs and calves. On the same day each month, I need you to go measure those same places and chart your progress. Nothing feels so great as to when you notice you have lost inches in one or more of those places. I am asking you to do this because we can't see our progress in the mirror most of the time and sometimes your weight doesn't show progress either. By measuring yourself you can see changes and celebrate those changes.

Weigh ins are not great sometimes. I want you to do them when you measure yourself though. Keep this log going and remember to keep your mind open to how much weight you want to lose because the number you have in your head may be different from when you decide you look and feel great. Also by staying on a healthy diet your weight could continue to drop without you trying. This is the bonus phase!

Chapter 6:
Exercise

I love exercise it make me feel wonderful but there are a few things you need to know. First of all, if you want to lose weight you need to be friends with some cardio. Now I don't need you to get on the treadmill for 6 hours and wear yourself ragged. To build muscle you need to do weights.

So here's the thing, you can work your butt off at the gym but if you are not watching what you eat you are wasting your time. So what do you need to do? Well you need to put 80% of your effort into the food you are eating. Make sure you are eating healthy food and real food. Then you need to put 20% of your effort into your exercise. I want you to walk one mile a day. When that gets to be easy walk 1.5 miles a day. I also want you to lift weights, do squats whatever you can do to build muscle. When you build muscle it eats fat. A gym membership is not necessary. Walk around the block a few times and track your mileage, do squats or push-ups for building muscles.

Now you are eating healthy food and exercising. That's great! Now we need to talk about eating enough to fuel that exercise. If you are burning 600 calories and only eating 1500 a day that means that you are down to 900 calories to fuel your body for the rest of the day. This is not enough for you to get by for the entire day. Eat your 2000 calories, don't worry about the extra calories. Especially if you are going to the gym and working those calories off. So let's recap. You need to be eating well, getting enough calories to allow your body to function properly and exercising enough to build muscle and burn a few calories. Tell yourself this is not hard you just need to take a few steps to turn your life around. Also you need to make sure you are done eating 4 hours before bed. If you do not finish at least 4 hours before bed your food is not getting digested before you become inactive.

Chapter 7:
It's Not a Race

I once heard someone say, "Don't expect the weight to come off right away, it took years to put on, it will take a while to take off". I feel like it's important for you to understand that it is really important for you to take your time and realize that it's not a race. Honestly, the slower you lose weight the easier it is going to be to keep it off. The reasoning behind this is because the longer you take the longer you get use to eating healthier. Also it gives your skin time to keep up with your weight loss. When you lose weight quickly the elasticity in your skin doesn't have the time it needs to keep up with your weight loss and you end up with the sagging arms and neck that everyone who has lost a lot of weight hates. So this is where I tell you to stop getting so upset because you only lost a pound this week. Or if you didn't lose at all, remember that it is ok and next week will be better. Take it slow this is not a race.

Chapter 8:
Recipes:

Well I can't give you a book without some helpful recipes to help you out with your new weight loss journey. I am going to give you recipes for Breakfast, lunch, dinner, sides and snacks so that you have options. You don't have to use these recipes in order to follow my diet plan, they are just simple helpful recipes for you to take advantage of. I feel like if I am sitting here telling you to eat healthy and stay away from certain things I really should be giving you items that you can eat in order to get excited about your new body. I also want you to realize that I don't want you to lose a bunch of weight and that's it. If you want to lose weight that is wonderful and this is the place to start. My main goal is to have a healthy you. I want you to feel good inside and out. It doesn't matter what that number on a scale says if you are feeling horrible.

Breakfast

Table of contents:

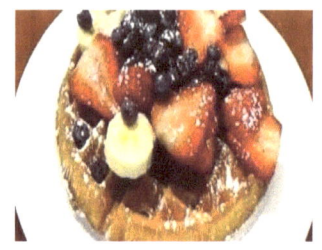

Buttermilk Waffles

With Fresh Fruit

Ingredients:
1 cup unbleached flour or whole wheat flour
¾ cup old-fashioned oats
1 Tbl baking powder
1 tsp baking soda
1 tsp salt
2 Tbl sugar
3 Tbl coconut oil
1 ¼ cups buttermilk
½ cup water
1 large egg
1 tsp vanilla
Fresh fruit I prefer sliced strawberries and blueberries) (Peaches also work well)
¼ tsp Powdered sugar

Directions:
Plug in your waffle iron. Combine first 6 ingredients in a large bowl. In a separate bowl combine your coconut oil, buttermilk, water, egg and vanilla. Once your liquid mixture is combined completely, slowly add your dry mixture and mix well.
Make sure your waffle iron is hot. Coat it with cooking spray to make sure it your batter doesn't stick. Pour your waffle batter into your iron, about ½ cup maybe a little more. Cook until it is golden brown. When you are done, place your waffle on a plate and then add your sliced fruit on top. Sprinkle your powdered sugar on top.

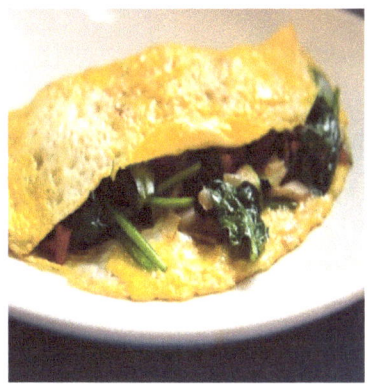

Vegetable Omelet

Ingredients:
1 tsp bacon grease (I use bacon grease because it is natural)
1 Tbl thinly sliced onion
3 Tbl chopped bell pepper (I like the red for its flavor)
½ cup Chopped baby spinach
3 cherry tomatoes diced
salt and pepper to taste
3 eggs beaten

Directions:
Heat half of your grease in a large nonstick pan. Cook your, onion, bell pepper, baby spinach and cherry tomatoes until cooked through. Be careful not to burn these.
Set your vegetables aside in a small bowl.
Add the remainder of your grease into your pan and heat. In a small bowl beat your eggs and add your salt and pepper to taste. Pour your eggs into your pan and let them cook for a good 30 seconds. Lift the edges of your eggs off the pan so that uncooked eggs can run under and begin to cook that also.
Once all of your eggs are cooked start adding in your vegetables to one side. You can also sprinkle some cheese in at this point.
Carefully fold over your eggs and place them on your plate. This omelet is two servings.

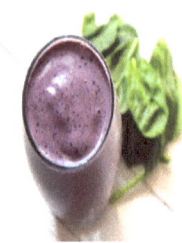

Banana Blueberry Smoothie

Ingredients:
2 frozen ripe bananas
½ cup frozen Blueberries
1 tsp honey
1 tsp vanilla
½ cup baby spinach
1 ½ cups Unsweetened almond milk (you may need more depending on how thin you like it)

Directions:
In your blender add your frozen bananas, honey and half of your almond milk. Turn on high until bananas are blended. Add the remainder of your ingredients and blend well. This should make about 4 servings. I use 6 ounce cups and feed this to my kids for an extra boost in the morning along with their breakfast.

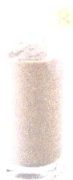

Peanut Butter Banana Smoothie

Ingredients:

1 Tbl Peanut butter
1 tsp honey
1 tsp vanilla
2 Frozen ripe bananas
1 ½ cups unsweetened almond milk

Directions:

In your blender add your frozen bananas, honey and half of your almond milk. Turn on high until bananas are blended. Add in the rest of your ingredients. You may need a little more almond milk in order for it to be thin enough.

This recipe makes a little less so I usually only get 2 to 3 servings of this one.

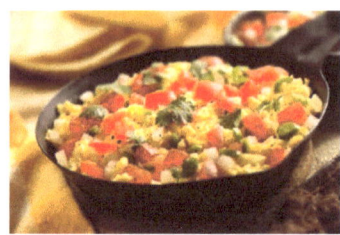

Vegetable Egg Scramble

Ingredients:

4 eggs
½ cup chopped baby spinach
¼ cup chopped onion
Chopped ham (thick slicked from the deli) Use the real stuff not processed!
3 cherry tomatoes chopped

Directions:

In a large pan on medium heat add your ham and vegetables. Cook until ham is warm and vegetables are cooked through. Add in your eggs and mix everything up while you are cooking it. Once everything is cooked through, throw it on a plate and enjoy.
I feed my family of 4 on this. Don't be scared off from all of the spinach, the way I cook you can't taste it and you get the benefits of the vitamins.

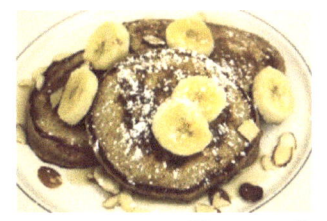

Banana nut Pancakes

Ingredients:

1 c. unbleached all-purpose flour

1 Tbl. sugar

2½ tsp. baking powder

½ tsp. salt

1¼ c. almond milk

2 Tbl. coconut oil

1 large egg

2 very ripe bananas

½ cup chopped walnuts

1 tsp banana extract

1 tsp vanilla extract

Directions

In a large bowl, with wire whisk, stir flour, sugar, baking powder, and salt. Add almond milk, coconut oil, and egg and stir until flour is moistened. Add your bananas and extracts then blend. Finally add in your walnuts and mix well.

Heat griddle or 12-inch skillet over medium heat. Pour batter onto your hot surface with a large ladle, making a few pancakes at a time. Cook until tops begin to bubble and edges begin to get dry. With a spatula, flip your pancake and continue cooking until golden brown. Transfer to a plate or platter and keep warm. I put mine in the microwave while waiting.

Continue until done with your batter.

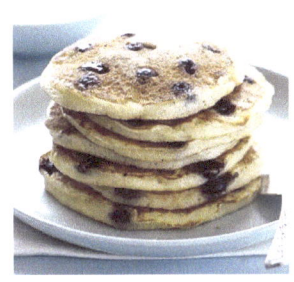

Blueberry Pancakes

Ingredients:

2 cups unbleached flour
1/3 cup sugar
2 Tbl baking powder
½ tsp salt
2 cups almond milk
2 eggs
1 tsp coconut oil
½ cup blueberries
1 tsp vanilla extract

Directions:

In a large bowl whisk together flour, sugar, baking powder and salt.
In a separate bowl whisk together milk, egg, oil and extract.
Add your dry and wet ingredients together and mix until just blended. Add your blueberries and fold in.
Spray a nonstick griddle and begin ladling on pancakes. Cook until bubbles start forming and your edges are dry. Turn your pancakes over and cook until golden brown. Place on a plate and keep warm until all of your pancakes are done.

Lunch

Table of contents:

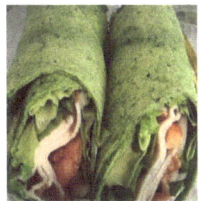

Spinach Turkey Wrap

Ingredients:

Sliced Turkey from the deli 2-3 slices
Baby spinach about ¼ cup
Bread and butter pickles 5-6 pickles
Spinach wrap
Shredded Lettuce
Shredded carrots
Italian salad dressing (1 Tbl)
Sliced avocado

Directions:

I like to heat up my tortilla. Lay your tortilla out on a plate place
everything in your tortilla and then fold he bottom up before folding
in the two sides.
This lunch has plenty of flavors and is oh so healthy.

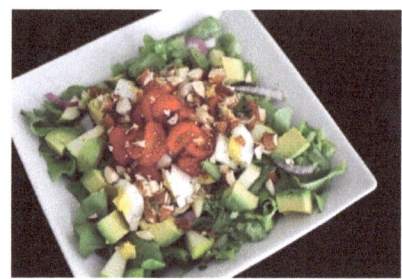

Loaded Salad

Ingredients:

1 cup of chopped lettuce
½ cup chopped baby spinach
1-2 slices of your favorite lunchmeat chopped
3-4 cherry tomatoes chopped
3-4 sliced black olives
1 hard-boiled egg chopped

Directions:

While you are chopping up all of your items boil one egg for 12 minutes. Throw everything together and enjoy with your favorite dressing.
Just because you are trying to lose weight does not mean you need to just eat lettuce. Enjoy your meal and add what you want to your salads.

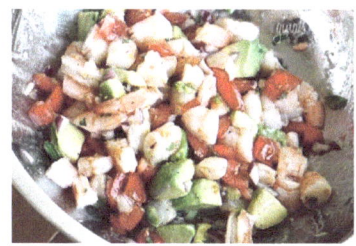

Shrimp Avocado Salad

Ingredients:

¼ cup chopped purple onion
2 limes (juiced)
1 tsp olive oil
¼ kosher salt, black pepper to taste
1 cup chopped baby spinach
1 lb jumbo cooked, peeled shrimp, chopped
1 Roma tomato diced
1 medium Hass avocado diced
1 Tbl chopped cilantro

Directions:

In a small bowl add your onion, limejuice, olive oil, salt and pepper. Let these marinate for 15 minutes.
In a separate bowl add your shrimp, avocado, baby spinach, tomato. Once you mix these add in your cilantro and mix it in. Now add in your onion mixture and salt and pepper to taste.

This recipe is so refreshing. It works really well on a hot day in Texas, is super healthy for you and is only 197 calories for a cup of the salad. I have to be honest; I probably eat at least two cups of this in one sitting.

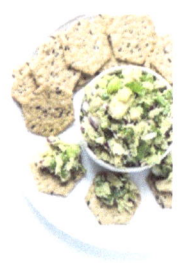

Tuna Salad with Crackers

Ingredients:

1 can of Tuna in water
¼ cup diced onion
1 tsp of fresh lemon juice
2 tsp extra virgin olive oil
¼ cup chopped parsley
½ avocado
½ tsp salt
¼ tsp pepper
5 saltine crackers

Directions:

You will need to add all of these things in a medium sized bowl.
You will notice there is no mustard or mayonnaise in this tuna salad.
Mayonnaise has a lot of fat in it so I try to use as little as possible.
Putting a cup of mayonnaise in your tuna is just bad for you. This
one will be creamy without the mayonnaise because of the Avocado.

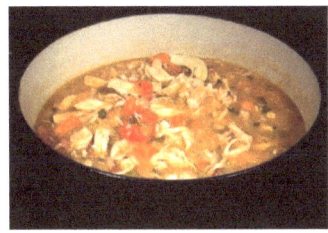

Mexican Chicken Soup

Ingredients:

Organic Black Beans 15oz. can (wash and drain)
1 can of corn or 2 ears of corn (drained)
1 Tbl. cilantro
1 can Rotel (drained)
30 oz. chicken broth
½ tsp paprika
½ tsp pepper
1 tsp sea salt
¼ tsp Cumin
2 lbs Chicken Breast

Directions:

Take all of your ingredients and place it in the Crockpot. Cover and let cook on low for 6 hours or put it in a large pot on the stove and cook for 1 hour.
This recipe can't get any easier and is delicious.

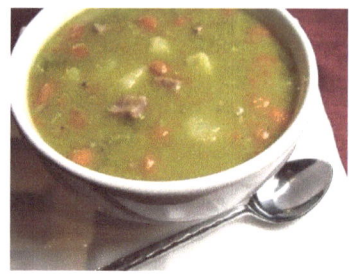

Split Pea Soup

Ingredients:

1 pound of chopped Ham (leftover or from the deli)
1 Bay leaf
2 carrots chopped
1 celery rib chopped
1 Tbl minced garlic
¼ cup parsley
1 16oz. bag of split peas. (I buy mine in the freezer section)
1 Tbl Thyme (I use fresh from the produce section)
½ cup white onion chopped
6 cups chicken broth
1 Tbl pepper
1 Tbl salt

Directions:

Wash all of your vegetable. In a large Crockpot place all of your ingredients except the chicken broth into you slow cooker once they are all chopped up. Add half of your chicken broth right now. Turn your Crockpot on and cook slowly for 7 to 8 hours. Each time you check your soup add a little bit more broth to it so that it doesn't dry up and you get more of a soup at the end.

Dinner

Table of contents:

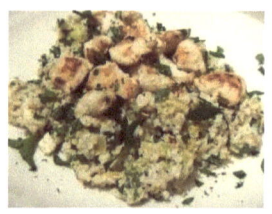

Creamy chicken and rice

Ingredients:

Chicken breasts

1 ½ cups uncooked rice

1 can chicken broth

1 carrot chopped

1 cup chopped baby spinach

3 large mushrooms diced

2 Tbl lime juice

1 tsp cayenne pepper

1 tsp salt

1 tsp pepper

1/8 cup almond milk original flavor

Directions:

I use a cast iron pan, if you do not make sure you have a large pan that is non-stick. Salt and pepper your chicken breasts and place them in the pan browning both sides.

Pour half the can of chicken broth in the pan with the chicken and pour the rice in with it.

Add all of your vegetables and pour the lime juice over the top.

You will slowly add the rest of your chicken broth as it cooks down. When you are done with that, slowly add water. I think I ended up adding a cup after all was set and done. Just let it cook down and add more until your rice is done. Sprinkle the cayenne pepper on top and mix in as you cook.

Just before everything is done add in 1/8 cup almond milk and let simmer for 3 minutes longer.

Serve with the rice and vegetable on bottom and the chicken on top. Super yummy.

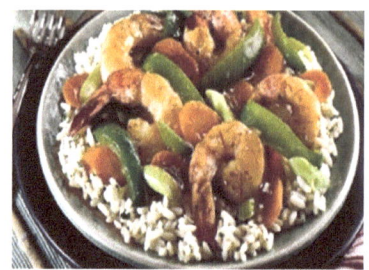

Stir-fry

Ingredients:

1-pound Uncooked Large shrimp
1 cup snap peas
1 cup red bell pepper chopped
½ cup white onion chopped
1 ½ cups chicken stock
3 Tbl cornstarch
1 Tbl soy sauce
½ tsp sesame oil
1/2 tsp garlic powder
3 cups cooked Jasmine rice

Directions:

I know it says cooked rice above but I wanted to note I usually start my rice before I do my stir-fry in a rice cooker. 1 ½ cups uncooked rice to 3 cups water.

In a large wok heat 1 Tbl of olive oil. Add your shrimp and cook through. Set aside.

Stir in your cornstarch, stock soy sauce and sesame oil in a small bowl.

In your wok add 1 Tbl of olive oil and add your vegetables and garlic powder. Stir-fry until your vegetables are tender-crisp. Add your cornstarch mixture to your vegetables and cook until it bubbles. Add your shrimp to your vegetables until warmed through and serve over your rice.

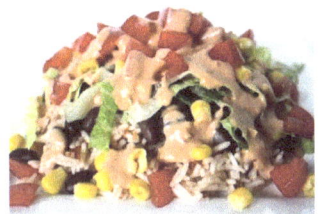

Burrito Bowl

Ingredients:

1 ½ cups cooked Jasmine Rice
3 uncooked chicken breasts
2 tsp lime juice
3 Tbl fajita seasoning
1 can drained and rinsed black beans
1 can drained and rinsed corn
1 head romaine lettuce washed and shredded
1 cup cherry tomatoes diced
½ cup ranch dressing
3 tsp Franks red hot sauce

Directions:

Take your chicken breasts and cut into 1 inch cubes. Place in a gallon sized Ziploc bag and add in your limejuice and fajita seasoning. Put this in the fridge to marinate for at least 15 minutes. I like to do mine for an hour. Once it is marinated throw it in a pan and cook through.
While that is cooking Take all of your vegetables and put them in separate bowls so that they are ready.
In a small bowl mix your ranch and hot sauce together.
When everything is done on your plate or in a bowl which ever you prefer layer, rice, lettuce, black beans, corn, tomatoes, fajita chicken and finally your sauce.

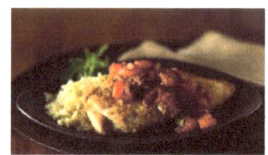

Tomato chicken

Ingredients:

4 Boneless skinless Chicken Breast
½ cup Progresso Panko Crispy Bread Crumbs
¼ cup fresh grated Parmesan cheese
½ tsp Salt
¼ tsp Pepper
3 Tbl olive oil
3 Large tomatoes chopped
2 medium green onions chopped
1 clove of garlic finely chopped
1 Tbl balsamic vinegar
1 Tbl chopped fresh oregano leaves

Directions:

Take your chicken Breasts and pound with the soft side of a mallet between wax paper as to cut down on messiness. Pound until about ¼ inch thick.
In a pie plate, add breadcrumbs, Parmesan, salt and pepper. Mix well. Coat each chicken breast with your mixture making sure to push the chicken down into it.
In a large non-stick pan, heat 2 Tbl olive oil over medium heat. Cook your chicken in the oil until cooked through and golden brown on both side flipping once. Remove chicken and cover to keep warm.
In the same pan add 1 Tbl olive oil, 2 cups of the tomatoes, onions, and garlic. Cook 2 minutes. Stir in Vinegar, cook 30 seconds.
Remove from heat. Stir in remaining tomatoes and oregano with the mixture you just removed from the pan.
Serve over your chicken.

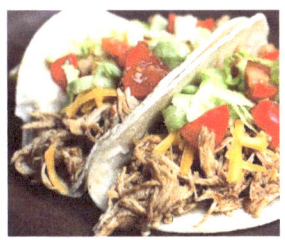

Chicken Tacos

Ingredients:

3 Frozen Chicken Breasts
1 package of chicken taco seasoning
1 can rotel
¼ cup olive oil
¼ cup water
Tortillas
Shredded lettuce
Diced tomatoes

Directions:

Add all of your ingredients to your Crockpot. Cook 4 ½ hours on low. Shred your chicken and return to Crockpot for another 30 minutes.
Serve on tortillas with shredded lettuce, avocado and tomatoes.

Side Note: You can also make this with pork. Just substitute pork tenderloin with your chicken and green enchilada sauce for the Rotel. There you go 2 meals one recipe!

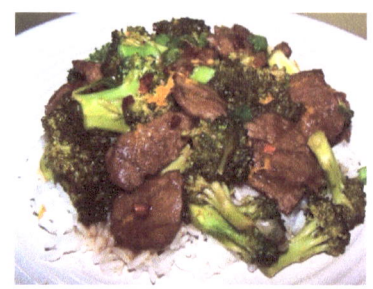

Orange Beef and Broccoli

Ingredients:

1 head of Broccoli
1/3 cup of Beef Broth
1/3 cup low-sugar orange marmalade
2 Tbl soy sauce
¼ tsp salt
2 Tbl cornstarch
1 lb. flank steak, cut into thin slices
1 Tbl red pepper flakes
3 cups cooked Jasmine Rice

Directions:

Cook your broccoli until it is still a little crisp.
While Broccoli is cooking, combine broth, marmalade, soy sauce and salt in a small bowl, stirring with a whisk and then set aside.
Put your cornstarch in a pie plate and drag your steak through it.
Heat a large nonstick skillet, coat with nonstick spray and add your steak. Cook for 5 minutes until brown. Add your broth and pepper flakes and cook for 1 minute making sure your sauce is thickening. Stir in your broccoli and serve immediately over your rice.

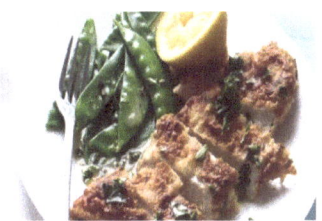

Lemon Chicken with Snow Peas

Ingredients:

1 10 oz package of frozen snow peas
2 eggs
¼ cup fresh grated Parmesan cheese
¼ cup chopped parsley
½ cup chicken broth
¼ cup lemon juice
½ tsp salt
¼ tsp pepper
4 skinless boneless chicken breasts, pounded to ¼ inch thick
¼ cup all-purpose flour (I use unbleached)
2 garlic cloves chopped
2 Tbl olive oil
3 Tbl butter
1 lemon cut into wedges

Directions:

Microwave your snow peas according to the directions on the package.
In a large bowl beat your eggs. Add Parmesan, parsley, ¼ cup of broth, 2 Tbl lemon juice, salt and pepper. Coat your chicken in flour and then coat in your egg mixture.
In a large skillet sauté your garlic in oil over medium heat for about 30 seconds. Add your chicken and cook for 8-10 minutes. Remove and place on a plate.

In the same skillet melt your butter. Stir in ¼ cup broth, and 2 Tbl lemon juice. Bring this to a boil and cook for about 30 seconds. Pour this sauce over your chicken and serve with your snow peas and add a lemon wedge to each plate.

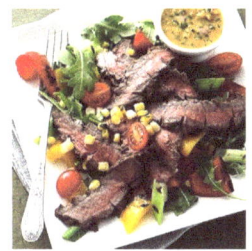

Grilled Flank Steak Salad with Roasted Corn Vinaigrette

Ingredients:

3 cups fresh corn kernels
½ cup chicken broth
2 Tbl lime juice
2 Tbl chopped red bell pepper
2 Tbl extra virgin olive oil
1 tsp salt
½ tsp pepper
½ cup chopped cilantro
1 Tbl cumin
2 tsp oregano dried
¼ tsp red pepper flakes
¾ lb. flank steak
1 Large head Romaine lettuce
4 cups halved cherry tomatoes
¾ cup sliced red onion
1/12 cups cooked black beans (can be canned but need to be drained and rinsed)

Directions:

In a large Cast iron or pan, add your corn and cook until it browns. This could take up to 5 minutes and then set aside in a bowl.

In a food processor add, stock, lime juice, bell pepper and 1 cup of your roasted corn. Pulse a few times and then add the olive oil, salt, pepper and cilantro. Pulse a couple times to blend and then set this aside. This will be your vinaigrette.

Heat a grill or broiler and coat with cooking spray. Make sure your cooking rack is away from your heat source directly. About 4-6 inches.

In a small bowl add your cumin, oregano, red pepper flakes and ½ tsp salt and ¼ tsp pepper. Rub this mixture on both sides of your steak.

Place your steak on your pre-heated grill or broiler and grill for 4-5 minutes on each side of your steak. Let stand for 5 minutes and then cut across the grain into this slices about 2 inches thick.

In a large bowl add your lettuce, tomatoes, onion, black beans, remaining roasted corn and your vinaigrette then toss to mix well. Serve your salad on a plate and then top with slices of your flank steak.

You can also top this with a few crumbles of Goat cheese for extra flavor.

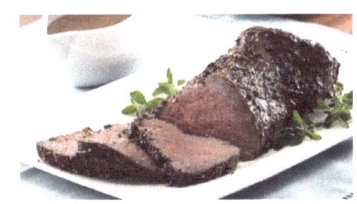

Peppered Roast Tenderloin

Ingredients:

1 2 ½ lb. Beef Tenderloin, trimmed and tied
2 garlic cloves, thinly sliced
4 tsp. Extra virgin olive oil
1 Tbl. Black pepper corn.
2 tsp finely chopped fresh rosemary
2 tsp finely chopped fresh thyme
2 tsp finely chopped fresh sage
½ tsp salt

Directions:

Pre-heat your oven to 425 degrees
With a small knife, slice small incisions all around the tenderloin.
Place garlic into each of your cuts and rub oil all over your
tenderloin. Mix together your spices and rub all over your tenderloin
making sure to rub it into the meat.
Place your meat into a roasting pan and roast for 10 minutes. Then
reduce your temp to 350 and roast until the internal temperature
reads 145 degrees. If you would like it more medium cook another
20 minutes. Transfer to a cutting board and let it rest for 15 minutes.
After your rest time slice into thin slices about ¼ inch thick.

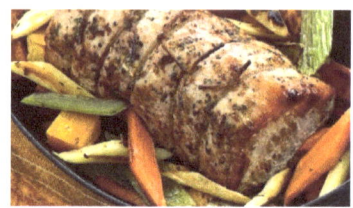

Pork Roast with Winter Vegetables

Ingredients:
2 large garlic cloves minced
zest of 1 lemon
1 Tbl. Chopped fresh rosemary
1 ½ tsp salt
½ tsp black pepper
1 2-pound boneless pork loin roast trimmed
½ butternut squash, peeled, seeded and cut into 1 inch cubes
3 large carrots peeled and sliced
4 celery stalks chopped
3 tsp extra virgin olive oil.

Directions:

Preheat your oven to 450 degrees. Spray a large roasting pan with nonstick spray.
Mix together your garlic, lemon zest, rosemary, salt and pepper and rub into your pork. Place pork into roasting pan. Arrange all of your veggies around your pork loin and season with salt and pepper.
Roast until a thermometer inserted into the middle reads 160 degrees. This usually takes about 45 minutes.
Place your pork on a cutting board and let it rest for 15 minutes.
Slice into ¼ inch slices and serve with your vegetables.
Side Note: I also squeeze lemon juice over the vegetables to give them a little extra flavor.

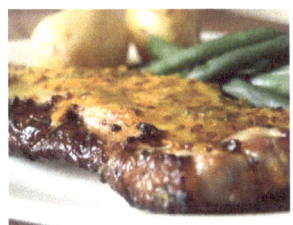

Honey Mustard Pork Chops

Ingredients:
1/3 cup Dijon mustard
4 tsp honey
1 tsp apple cider vinegar
¼ tsp black pepper
1 tsp sea salt
4 bone in pork chops

Directions:

In a small bowl add all of your ingredients except the chops.
Place your pork chops in a gallon size zip lock and pour your
marinade in over it.
Squeeze out all of your air and zip closed. Place in the fridge to
marinade for at least 4 hours. I do mine overnight.
Spray broiler rack with nonstick spray and place your chops on the
rack. Broil 5 inches from the heat for 6 minutes on each side.

Notes:
This is perfect for getting together the night before or in the morning
before work. When you get home from work it takes 15 minutes to
cook.

Snacks

Table of Contents:

Frozen Grapes

Frozen grapes are my favorite snack right now. I know it's something little and something easy but it is quick and when you are trying to not eat popsicles they are a perfect substitute.

Wash your favorite grapes, put them in a snack sized Ziploc baggie and throw them in the freezer. They will be good for up to 3 months and are perfect to stop that wonderful sugar craving you are having.

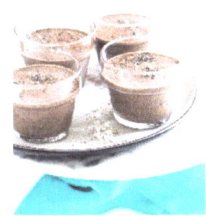

Chocolate Vanilla Chia Pudding

Ingredients:

1 1/2 cups Almond Breeze Unsweetened

1/3 cup chia seeds

1/4 cup unsweetened cocoa powder

1/2 tsp ground cinnamon

1/2 tsp vanilla extract

Directions:

Add all of your ingredients into a medium sized cup and mix well. Place it in the fridge for at least 4 hours but it does best when it sets overnight. You can also add sliced bananas, strawberries or blueberries on top.

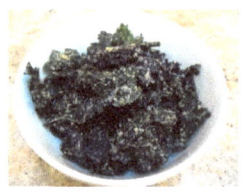

Zesty kale chips

Ingredients:

1 bunch of Kale washed and dried
Extra virgin Olive Oil
Sea Salt
Seasoning salt

Directions:

Preheat over to 350 degrees
Tare your kale leaves into bite size pieces.
In a large bowl sprinkle about 1 Tbl olive oil on top of the kale. Toss to coat then sprinkle salt and seasoning salt on your kale and toss again.
Place your kale in a single layer on a baking sheet that has been lined with parchment paper.
Bake for 12-14 minutes or until they are crisp. Half way through toss them around on the baking sheet to make sure everything cooks evenly and you don't get any burnt edges.
You can also do variances, garlic salt or powder, chili flakes or really any seasoning you just can't get enough of.

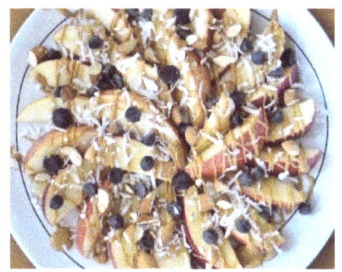

Apple Nachos

Ingredients:

1 apple (your favorite kind)
Peanut butter
1/8 cup Coconut
1/8 cup Walnuts
1/8 cup Mini chocolate chips
Honey

Directions:

Take your apple and slice it into thin slices. Thick enough for them not to bend when you pick them up.
Spread on a thin layer of Peanut butter.
In a food processor, add your coconut, walnuts and chocolate chips. Pulse until your chocolate chips have been chopped up a bit and you can sprinkle the mixture.
Take your mixture and sprinkle everything on top of the apple slices. You may have some left over.
Drizzle honey over the top of your Nachos.

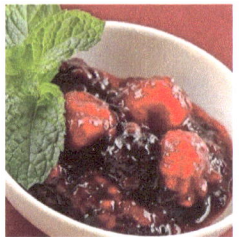

Fresh Berries with Ginger Sauce

Ingredients:

4 cups strawberries
¼ cup fresh orange juice
3 Tbl chopped crystallized ginger
½ tsp vanilla extract
2 cups blackberries
1 cup raspberries
fresh mint leaves

Directions:

In a blender add your strawberries, orange juice, ginger and vanilla and blend until smooth.
Strain your juice into a bowl. Press on the solids in order to get out all of the juice.
In a large bowl, add your blackberries, and raspberries and toss them together.
In small serving bowls add some frit and spoon some of your sauce over it. Add your mint to garnish your fruit and serve immediately.

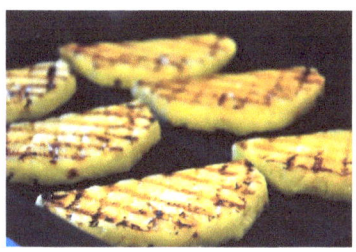

Grilled Pineapple

Ingredients:

1 fresh pineapple
3 Tbl honey
1 Tbl limejuice
½ tsp seasoning salt

Directions:

Trim your pineapple and cut into slices.
In a bowl add your honey and seasonings and mix well.
Brush your sauce on your pineapple
Pre-heat your grill and spray with nonstick spray.
Grill your pineapple for 4 minutes on each side. Do not overcook or your pineapple or it will turn mushy. Be careful not to burn your pineapple.

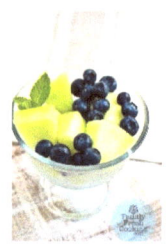

Fruit Salad with Lime and Mint

Ingredients:

1 cup honey dew melon
¾ cup blueberries
¼ Tbl. Chopped fresh mint
½ Tbl fresh lime juice

Directions:

Place all of your ingredients into a medium-mixing bowl and toss everything together. Set in the fridge to chill for about an hour. Serve cold.

Sides

Table of contents:

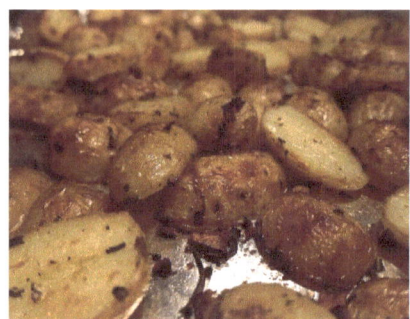

Rosemary lime new potatoes

Ingredients:

5 large white potatoes
1 Tbl extra virgin olive oil
2 tsp rosemary
2 tsp sea salt
1 tsp pepper
1 tablespoon lime juice

Directions:

Heat your oil in a large on-stick pan.
Wash and chop your potatoes into small cubes and throw them into
your pan.
Season your potatoes as you are cooking them and make sure to
cook them all the way through.
Add your lime juice and cook 1 more minute.

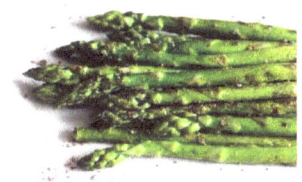

Grilled asparagus

Ingredients:

1 bunch of Asparagus washed and trimmed (cut off the bottom part about an inch up.)
Extra virgin olive oil
Salt
Pepper
Garlic Powder

Directions:

After you have washed and trimmed your Asparagus dry it off with paper towels.
Lay your asparagus on a flat surface and with a basting brush, brush olive oil onto your asparagus.
Sprinkle salt, pepper and garlic powder to taste.
On a grill or in a cast iron pan lay your Asparagus in a single layer and heat on high until cooked through. This usually takes about 2-3 minutes on the grill and about 4-5 in a cast iron.

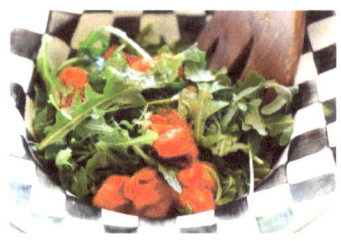

Side salad with sundried tomatoes

Ingredients:

½ cup sun dried tomatoes
1 head of Romaine Lettuce
1 small cucumber
1/8 cup chopped Black olives
2 banana peppers
Homemade Italian dressing

Directions:

For your sun dried Tomatoes:
Pre-heat your oven to 200 degrees
Wash and halve 1 cup of cherry tomatoes. I squeeze out the seeds.
Put your tomatoes on a cookie sheet and season with Italian seasonings.
Bake until they are dried out and resemble a leathery texture. Mine usually takes about 4 hours.

For your salad:
Chop up all of your ingredients except your tomatoes and throw them in a large bowl.
Toss your salad to mix up all of your ingredients.
Put your tomatoes on top and then make your salad dressing.

For your dressing:
Whisk together, ¼ cup white vinegar, 2/3 cup extra virgin olive oil, 2 tablespoons of water.
When this is blended add.

1/8 tsp garlic salt
1/8 tsp onion powder
¼ tsp dried oregano
pinch of pepper
pinch of thyme
pinch of dried basil
pinch of dried parsley
¼ tsp fine sea salt
Whisk together all of the ingredients with your wet mixture until blended well.

Add your dressing to the entire salad and toss or set it on the table so that each person can use as much as they want.

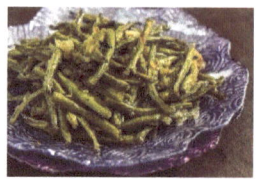

Fresh garlic and onion green beans

Ingredients:

Fresh green beans cleaned and chopped (I use about 2 cups)
2 Tbl minced garlic
½ red onion in thin slices
2 tsp fine sea salt
¼ cup chicken stock

Directions:

In a large stockpot add your chicken stock and onions on medium heat.
While your onions are cooking chop your green beans. Cut the ends off and cut in half. Throw this into your pot with your onions. Cook this for about 5 minutes.
Add in your garlic and sea salt and cook until your green beans are cooked to your desired tenderness. I usually cook mine for a total of 20 minutes. Make sure you are watching your beans and stirring them occasionally so that they do not burn.

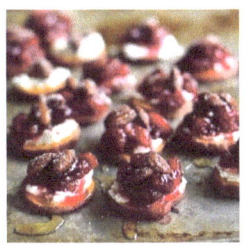

Sweet Potato Rounds with Goat Cheese

Ingredients:

2 large sweet potatoes
2 Tbl melted butter
4 Tbl Goad cheese
Dried Cranberries
Toasted pecans

Directions:

Preheat your oven to 450 degrees.
Wash your sweet potatoes and cut into slices about ¼ inch thick.
Lightly brush your potatoes with your melted butter and place in a
9x13 glass pan. Bake these for 20 minutes or until done making sure
to turn them half way through your cooking process.
Once they are done cooking take them out of the pan and place them
on a paper towel to get your oil off.
Take 3 to 4 pieces of your potatoes and out them in a plate and top
with 1 Tbl goat cheese a couple of cranberries and some toasted
pecans.

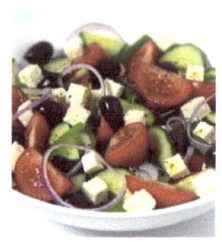

Greek Salad

Ingredients:

1 head of Romaine Lettuce
½ red onion sliced thin
½ cup black olives
1 red bell pepper chopped
10 cherry tomatoes quartered
1 small cucumber
½ cup feta cheese

Directions:

Chop up all of your veggies and add to a large bowl.

For your dressing:
Whisk together 6 Tbl extra virgin olive oil, 1 tsp dried oregano, 1 lemon juiced, and ground pepper to taste.
Pour over your salad and toss to mix well.

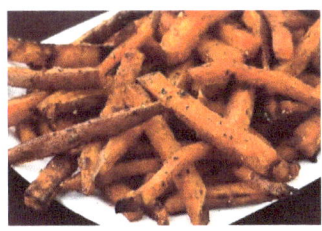

Sweet Potato Fries

Ingredients:

2 Medium sweet potatoes
1 Tbl extra virgin olive oil
¼ tsp sea salt
½ tsp paprika

Directions:

Take your sweet potatoes and wash them and scrub them.
Heat your oven to 425 degrees
Slice your potatoes lengthwise into 8 pieces.
In a gallon size Ziploc toss your potatoes, oil and seasonings together to coat.
Put your potatoes on a baking sheet in a single layer.
Cook for about 15 minutes or until lightly browned n the bottoms.
Turn your potatoes over and bake for another 10 minutes or until the bottom is browned again.
Serve hot and try not to put Ketchup all over them. If you need to though keep it at a minimum.

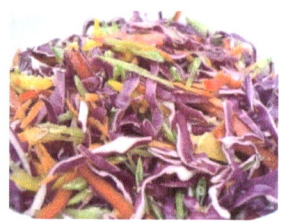

Rainbow Slaw

Ingredients:

For slaw:
2 cups shredded green cabbage
½ cup shredded or grated carrot
½ cup shredded red cabbage
¼ cup red onion sliced thin
For dressing:
½ avocado
¼ cup filtered water (add slowly)
2 tablespoons apple cider vinegar
1 Tbl Dijon mustard
1 tsp minced garlic
1 tsp sea salt
1/8 tsp black pepper

Directions:

Shred all of your vegetables and add to a large bowl.
In a blender add all of your ingredients for your dressing with the exception of the water. Blend your ingredients and slowly add your water until smooth and at the thickness you prefer it. Pour into your bowl with your slaw and mix well. You can serve this at room temp or chill it in your fridge before serving.

Chapter 9:
Extra tips and information

So now that you have read the information and seen the recipes I figured I would let you know a few more things that I feel you might need know about my weight loss. Things like, why you can eat certain things and why you shouldn't. First of all, I suffer from Lactose intolerance and IBS. I have to be on a strict diet or I get sick. This is a huge pain when I go out to eat or over to others houses to eat. However, in saying that, I don't have slip ups because I get sick from those. That makes me going on a diet a little easier. If you want to drop some weight, I have given you the tools to do it. The problem is you are going to have to be strict with yourself.

Why we have rice- Rice is known to be a filler, something that keeps you full and expands in your stomach. As with everything you are putting in your body making sure you don't eat too much is key. Keep things to a minimum and don't overdo it.

Lack of milk- You may have noticed the lack of milk or dairy products. As I mentioned above I am lactose intolerant. The lack of those fats could have something to do with some of my weight loss. This is also why in most of my recipes I don't have any milk and very little dairy. I am trying to give you the tools you need in order to get where you want to be in life. You want to lose weight, cut the sugar and if you feel the need cut the dairy cut that also. I am not saying it won't help because I am sure it will, but this one is up to you.

Lack of cheese and processed items- Cheese goes along with the whole no dairy thing. In my bad fats list in the beginning of the book I mentioned cheese as a bad fat. This isn't going to change just because it tastes good. I will say some cheese is not bad; again just don't overdo it. If you choose to eat cheese go to the deli and get the real stuff. I know it is more expensive, but it is real. It is not something that has been filled with junk. In the beginning I told you get off the processed foods and most of your sugar. This includes processed cheese because it isn't real and you really need real food in your body that is easily digestible.

I'm going to finish off by going over all my rules to losing weight one more time.

Get off as much sugar as you can.

Do not eat anything that says sugar free

Instead look for things that say No Sugar Added

Eat healthy fats

Give up all of the processed foods

Eat as many leafy greens as you can every single day

Cut back on the dairy if you feel lit will give you an extra edge

Drink your water

Season your food so it actually tastes good!

Do your meal plan each week so you have less chance of slip ups

Last and not least:

Do not get hard on yourself this will take time!